Men in Bras, Panties and Dresses

The Secret Truths about Transvestites

One in ten men regularly wears feminine clothing. Cross-dressers live longer, healthier lives than other men. But many wives and girlfriends don't know their man's undercover secrets.

Vernon Coleman

Published by the European Medical Journal
A European Medical Journal Special Monograph

The right of Vernon Coleman to be identified as the author of this work has been asserted in accordance with the Copyright, Designs and Patents Act 1988.
First edition published by the European Medical Journal in 1995. Revised edition published 2014.

ISBN:978-1-898947561

A catalogue record for this book is available from the British Library.

Table of Contents

'The transvestite is a man who has discovered a way of being at peace with herself. Transvestism is a gift not a curse; we should be grateful for it.'

Anonymous transvestite

Introduction

This European Medical Journal Special Monograph is based on a study of 1,015 British males. The study was conducted, and the report written, by Dr Vernon Coleman MB ChB DSc – a registered and licensed medical practitioner.

Abstract

There are many myths and misconceptions about why men cross dress. This survey shows quite clearly that most cross-dressers are neither homosexual nor aspirational transsexuals. Cross dressing is not an illness and most transvestites do not want to be 'cured'. Transvestism is regarded by many as a valuable remedy for stress. The variations among cross-dressers are vast. Some men like dressing entirely in female clothing; some enjoy wearing individual items of feminine apparel. Some go out in public dressed in female clothing while others stay indoors while cross-dressed. Some wear feminine lingerie underneath male clothing. Transvestism crosses all class and social barriers but seems to be exceptionally common among men who have acquired exceptional responsibilities.

Transvestism: A Social Phenomenon

It is doubtful if anyone knows exactly how many men obtain pleasure, sexual satisfaction or relief from stress by dressing up in women's clothes (or, more accurately, clothing designed primarily for women to wear). The potential embarrassment and perceived social stigma associated with transvestism means that many men are extremely secretive about their cross-dressing habits; consequently it is difficult to obtain an accurate figure. Some authorities have claimed that as many as 50% of men have, at some time or another, dressed partly or completely in women's clothes. More conservative estimates put the number regular transvestites at around 10% of the male population in most developed countries. It seems that cross dressing is currently one of the fastest growing social phenomena in the western world.

My own studies suggest that the figure of 1 in 10 is probably accurate. And that the figure is undoubtedly rising quite rapidly. It seems that cross dressing is currently one of the fastest growing social phenomena in the western world.

History

Cross-dressing isn't new, of course. Men and women have been doing it since clothing was invented. Transvestism occurs to some degree in the oldest societies, whether sophisticated or primitive.

In some societies, transvestites were ridiculed (as they usually are today) but far more often they were treated with respect, and regarded as possessing great wisdom and of having magical or mystical qualities. Christian saints and Hindu gods have changed sex at will and Hippocrates reported that men who dressed as women became priests. Ancient Jewish history contains accounts of men dressing as women. Caligula used to dress as a woman as did at least one English king and one French king. Today, shamans (powerful and deeply respected figures in religions around the world) are often men dressed in feminine clothing.

The most famous transvestite in history was probably Le Chevalier d'Eon de Beaumont, a lawyer, political adventurer, spy and diplomat in the service of Louis XV. He was born in 1728, christened Charles Genevieve Louise Auguste Andre Timothee d'Eon de Beaumont and died at the age of 82, having spent 48 years living as a man and 34 living as a woman. The word 'eonism' is now often used as a synonym for 'transvestism' or 'cross-dressing'.

Cross-dressing hasn't always involved men dressing in feminine clothing, of course. Female suffragettes in England often dressed as men and in the 18th century it was fairly common for Dutch women to dress as men in order to obtain work as sailors.

Part of the problem for transvestites is the fact that we are so wrapped up in what we now consider to be 'proper' or 'acceptable' behaviour that we often forget that fashion is never more than fleeting. In some cultures it is women who wear the trousers and men who wear the skirts. Painting finger nails is currently considered to be a feminine preserve but the habit originated in China where warriors going into battle would paint their nails crimson in the hope that this would give the enemy the impression that their hands were already dripping with blood.

Terminology

The words 'transvestite' and 'cross-dresser' are used throughout this monograph as though they were totally interchangeable: both referring to an individual (usually and in the case of this study exclusively male) who dresses in the clothes normally associated with the opposite sex. The word 'cross-dresser' is generally preferred by those heterosexuals who wish to establish a clear difference between themselves and others such as 'drag queens'. However, I have retained the word 'transvestite' since this is in general use. The terms 'cross-dresser' and 'transvestite' are usually regarded as referring to males who wear clothing normally associated with women, for the simple reason that cross-dressing among women (millions of whom regularly wear trousers, shirts, jackets and other items of clothing traditionally associated with men) is so commonplace that it is not regarded as in any way exceptional or worthy of comment. In some communities, indeed, it is more usual to see women wearing trousers than to see them wearing dresses or skirts.

The Survey: the form used

The transvestites who took part in the survey were invited to complete the following survey form:

1. How old were you when you first started wearing women's clothes?
2. Why do you do it? (tick as many of the options as you like)
a) I like the feeling of women's clothing
b) It gives me a sexual kick
c) It helps me relax and deal with stress
d) I want to be like a woman
e) I don't know
3. If you had the opportunity would you have a sex change operation? Yes/No
4. Do you dress completely as a woman (e.g. including wig, make up etc)? Yes/No
5. Has being a transvestite ever lost you
a) A job
b) A relationship
6. Do you go out of the house dressed as a woman? Yes/No
7. Do you attend parties, social events with other transvestites? Yes/No
8. Do you ever go shopping dressed as a woman? Yes/No
9. If you go out cross dressed, in your opinion, how many of the people who see you are convinced that you are a woman?
a) None
b) A few
c) Most
d) All
10. Do you wear women's underwear when you are dressed in ordinary male clothes?
a) Never
b) Occasionally
c) Always
11. What do you sleep in?
a) The nude
b) Pyjamas

c) Nightie

12. Have you ever had sex with another man? Yes/No

13. Do you live in fear of people finding out that you are a transvestite? Yes/No

14. Has cross dressing ever got you into trouble with the law? Yes/No

15. Have you ever had sex with a woman while you've been dressed as a woman? Yes/No

16. Does your partner know of your transvestism? Yes/No

17. Does she approve?

a) Not at all

b) With reluctance

c) With enthusiasm

18. Does your partner help you choose clothes, make up and so on? Yes/No

19. How many daytime hours a week do you spend dressed as a woman?

20. How many daytime hours a week would you like to spend dressed as a woman?

About yourself: (all optional – but please give as much information as you feel able)

Age:

Partner's Age:

Name:

Female name you use when dressed in feminine clothing:

Occupation:

Address:

The Survey: Results, Commentaries and Quotes from Cross-dressers

1. Survey Results: At what age do Cross-dressers Start Wearing Women's Clothing?

Question asked: How old were you when you began wearing women's clothes?

The average age at which males in this survey started dressing in women's clothes was 13. One individual reported that he had started cross-dressing at the age of four. The oldest respondent was 70 when he started dressing in feminine clothing.

Commentary

Transvestites who start young usually do so either because they are encouraged to do so by relatives or because they discover a tactile thrill from wearing clothes of a texture quite different to the clothes they normally wear. One bank manager reported that he regularly wore a lacy bra and panties and a garter belt and stockings underneath his three piece pinstriped suit simply because he liked the feel of the lingerie against his skin. Although some transvestism is actively encouraged (for example, by mothers who dress their sons as daughters – often because they wish they had given birth to a daughter rather than a son) there is often an element of secretiveness about 'cross dressing' right from the very beginning.

Transvestites who start cross dressing later in life often do so because they find their lives unbearably stressful and demanding and because they need to 'escape'; they need some form of release and discover that cross-dressing provides them with an opportunity to forget their male responsibilities.

Quotes from cross-dressers

'I was approximately eight or nine years old. My mother used to throw old clothes out for the "rag-bag" and I used to get them out and dress up in them. I graduated from there to raiding her drawers and wardrobe and from there to stealing items of clothing from female relatives when we went visiting. I became quite adept at asking to go to the toilet and taking a wrong turning into Aunty's bedroom to pinch a petticoat or a pair of knickers.'

'From about the age of four I've been hooked on wearing female underwear. At that early age I used to steal what I could from washing lines and sneak them into the house and put them on in front of the mirror and pose and wear them in heels and masturbate into them. It was great fun. I never got caught stealing them but gave that up as I thought that one day I might.'

'My earliest memory of dressing up was when I was four. I believe that my reasons for cross dressing started at this age. I can remember my late mother speaking to her friends and saying that she always wanted a daughter, to be called Ann, and when told at the nursing home that she had a boy she said that she didn't want him. I am not experienced in psychology but I think that must be the cause.'

'One of my earliest memories was when I was about seven years old and I saw a pair of my mother's tights in her room. Alongside them was a pair of blue court shoes. I went into her room, picked up the tights, gathered up the leg as I'd seen her do and I slowly slipped my foot inside its nylon sheath and began to gently and steadily roll it up to my calf toward my knee. Then I looked at my tights clad leg and something said to me that this was right. I then put on her shoes and felt the high heels hoist me to even greater desires.'

'The first time I became aware of female clothing and of its appeal, was as a small child when I was put to bed as a toddler in ladies' knickers because I had run out of night wear. I had a fever with German measles; all my clothes had become damp and were in the wash. I can still remember how I wished I could wear the same clothes the next night...without any idea why! But I can remember after all these years the yearning that a small child felt to wear silk knickers. This could hardly be a sexual need or kick, not as a little toddler!'

'The compulsion to wear female clothing began by chance at the age of 10. For no apparent reason I went into my sister's bedroom and finding her underwear drawer open, I took her bra and panties to my room and tried them on. She was coming up to her 12th birthday and had decided that only girls would be invited to her party. I had been pressing to be included for some time to no avail. Although I had returned the bra to the drawer, the panties were found in my room. I was told not to take other people's things again and I thought that was the end of the matter. Two weeks later on the day of the party I was told that they had changed their minds and I could go but they had a surprise for me. I was led to my bedroom and to my horror laid out on my bed was a party dress, frilly knickers, knee length white socks and even a 'Shirley Temple' type wig. Despite my protests I was told if I wanted to be a girl here's my chance. The party went ahead and I was the centre of fun. It did not end there. For two weeks every evening after school I had to change into girl's clothing as a punishment. To my surprise, as the evenings went on I found I was secretly enjoying the experience. Since then at every opportunity I have cross dressed. My relatives who had started me on this road are totally opposed to this idea of men dressing in women's clothing. In fact they think those who do it are 'sick'.'

'If I had no clean underwear, my mother used to put a pair of my sister's knickers on me. I used to get upset at first, but I grew to enjoy the feel of satin, lace, etc., and the pretty, frilly, fussy look of female underwear.'

'I spent a lot of time in one aunt's house who was a dressmaker. She used me as a model when making dresses when I stayed at her house.'

'It started when I was about nine or ten years old. As I was tubby I was always being ribbed about my breasts and about needing to wear a bra! I commenced by trying on corsetry and progressed to stockings, slips, panties and dresses and found I thoroughly enjoyed the experience.'

'I was a girl in various all-boys school dramatic society events (Cleopatra's handmaiden, a Welsh maid, Titania, a chorus girl in crinolines, and Juliet) before my voice broke; then I deputised as a girl in a couple of dance routines at about 14 years. I am sure this set a pattern, but after that it was too 'sissy' until after National Service. I made occasional forays in my early twenties (I used to go out with some nurses in Birmingham dressed as one of them). This went on for about a year, then in middle age I took it up seriously, first as a closet TV, and now openly with my wife's support.'

'I tried on a pair of my wife's panties one day. I was in my mid-fifties at the time. I have no idea why I did it. But it felt good. There was no looking back.'

'I started off just wearing my wife's knickers. I didn't think it would go any further than that. Then I started wearing a camisole top and then a bra. Eventually I started putting on a dress. By the time I got to that stage I realised I was a lost cause and that I might as well put make-up on as well. I then had to buy a wig so that I could go out of the house in my dress and make-up. A bald man walking down the street in a frock would look pretty stupid wouldn't he?'

2. Survey results: Why do Men Cross-dress?

Question asked: Why do you do it?

Note: Respondents were invited to tick as many options as they liked.

a) Because I like the feeling of women's clothes: 77%
b) Because it gives me a sexual kick: 59%
c) Because it helps me relax and deal with stress: 48%
d) Because I want to be like a woman: 63%

Commentary
It is clear that many transvestites dress for more than one reason.
Surprisingly, perhaps, the most common reason given for cross dressing was the feeling of wearing women's clothes. Men who are accustomed to wearing rough and itchy clothing obtain considerable tactile pleasure from contact with the thinner, softer, more delicate fabrics used in the manufacture of women's clothing. Although this feeling sometimes arises as a result of a childhood experience there

are many transvestites who have discovered the pleasure of wearing silky, satiny materials in their 30's, 40's or older. 'Putting on stockings for the first time was, without question, the single most erotic, sensually exciting thing I have ever done without a woman,' wrote one transvestite.

Many transvestites also report that they find cross dressing helps them deal with stress.

'Men dress for different reasons. I don't dress to shock or to be glamorous or sexy. I don't dress to attract men (or women). I don't do it for any reason other than to relax. Cross-dressing gets me out of myself. I don't want to be cured because there is nothing wrong with me. I won't ever stop.'

The twentieth century male is under a tremendous amount of pressure to be strong, masculine and successful. It is no coincidence that cross dressing is particularly popular among those men who are either workaholics or who are involved in particularly macho activities (such as the military or the police).

Transvestites who cross-dress to escape from stress are often workaholics. Having pushed themselves hard they are frequently successful in their business or professional careers and so they have a great deal to lose if their transvestism is exposed. Like all workaholics the transvestite workaholic pushes himself to the point of mental and physical exhaustion because he is searching for a love that has always been denied to him by his parents. Dressing as a woman enables him to escape completely from the pressure to succeed because it enables him to escape from his tortured male persona for a while.

A man who is under constant pressure to achieve, to perform and to make money may find that he can escape from those pressures most effectively by slipping on silky, feminine clothes. He can change his personality and his perception of society's expectations of him within seconds. He removes his suit or uniform and with it puts aside his responsibilities. When he puts on a pair of stockings, a garter belt and a dress or a skirt the soft, feminine side of his personality (which may have been suppressed for years) is allowed to come to the surface.

Time and time again, cross-dressers have told me that putting on a frock helps to bring out the gentle, non-aggressive, calm side of their personalities (the qualities which society wrong regards as 'feminine'.) Moreover, many cross-dressers have told me that they have never been able to find any other form of relaxation which is anywhere near as effective as cross-dressing in enabling them to step aside from the demands of their masculinity for a while; and to be more accepting, less demanding of themselves, more easy-going and more relaxed.

It is because cross-dressing is an effective way of dealing with stress and tension and pressure that many high flyers, politicians, military men, business leaders and professionals enjoy cross-dressing. There are an increasing number of clubs in the USA where business, political and military leaders can learn how to put on make-up, borrow clothing, relax and forget their everyday pressures and anxieties. In the UK male transvestites can now get a bank card to use when they are dressed as women.

One of the reasons why cross-dressing is so often done in secret is the fact that it is particularly common among the most successful men in business, the services and the professions – the very men who have most to lose by being 'found out' and who are, therefore, least likely to admit to cross dressing.

Many men who cross dress to escape from stress claim that when they put on stockings, a bra and a dress they can feel their cares and worries fading away. They feel calm and relaxed and so their bodies benefit enormously. Moreover, selecting and purchasing underwear, and putting on lipstick and nail varnish, helps them to find a different part of their personality and to forget their day to day anxieties. For them transvestism is a healthier way of relaxing than smoking or drinking and probably no more expensive or absurd a hobby than golf.

Cross dressing has no physical side effects (though there are still many social hazards – ranging from embarrassment through to unemployment). As a physician I would much rather see a man under stress deal with pressure by cross dressing than by taking tranquillisers.

Some may feel it surprising that anyone should be able to throw off stresses simply by putting on different clothes. But there is plenty of evidence to show that clothes do have an impact on the way we look at the world and the way we feel.

When a man dresses in his 'Sunday best' suit he will often feel and behave quite differently to the way he feels and behaves when

13

he is wearing his work or leisure clothes. Simply putting on a suit may affect the way he walks and talks – as well as the way he thinks. When I was a senior medical student and a young doctor I had a smart, pinstriped suit which I kept for important, formal occasions. I wore it mainly for examinations and for job interviews. Consequently, it was hardly surprising that I found myself feeling stressed and 'uptight' whenever I wore that suit. Eventually, just looking at the suit made me feel tense and so I gave it away to a charity shop knowing that the new owner would buy it without any emotional baggage.

In exactly the same way that my suit made me feel stressed so the transvestite can throw off his day to day worries – the worries normally associated with his male persona – and feel relaxed by taking off his working clothes (which he associates with anxiety) and putting on a dress (which is very different to the suit, uniform or working clothes he wears to work).

There are, without doubt, other ways in which a man under stress could obtain relief. But most of the available alternatives are likely to be considerably more damaging to him, his family and society in general than dressing up in fancy lingerie. The cross dresser could undoubtedly obtain a similar level of release by taking tranquillisers (likely to become an addictive habit), smoking cigarettes (likely to give him cancer) or drinking himself senseless.

Alcohol alters the senses and so makes stress bearable for many. Clothes can affect the senses with a similar result. The difference is that wearing silks and satins won't wreck your liver. (As an aside it is strange that the importance of the skin as a sense organ is so vastly and consistently underestimated.)

It seems odd that society should, in general, choose to regard alcoholism as a forgivable and understandable consequence of overwork, whereas cross dressing remains such a misunderstood remedy that most transvestites make enormous efforts to keep their dressing a secret.

(The secret nature of transvestism is something of a self-perpetuating problem: transvestites who are secretive inevitably risk being exposed and if they are exposed the fact that they kept their transvestism secret makes it sound as if even they consider it to be rather unpleasant habit. The fact that they kept it secret suggests to the observer that they were ashamed of it.)

Because of its importance in the relief of stress transvestism could, if promoted more actively, become one of the most important social developments of the century.

Many of the men who responded to my survey request were open about the fact that they get a sexual kick out of wearing women's clothes, though some pointed out that they merely enjoyed the erotic feeling of putting on feminine clothing. When you consider that feminine clothing is invariably much more erotic than the male equivalents (stockings to socks, camisoles to string vests, silky French knickers to Y front underpants) it is, perhaps, hardly surprising that some transvestites get a sexual kick out of dressing in feminine clothing. Some reported that cross-dressing helped to sexually stimulate themselves and their female partners. It is important to point out, however, that many cross-dressers do not believe there to be any sexual motive in their wearing of feminine clothing.

Medical and psychological textbooks sometimes claim that cross-dressing is a purely or largely sexual activity and this is clearly not true.

Quotes from cross-dressers
'I find painting my toe nails the most relaxing thing I've ever done. I have to concentrate but it takes no real effort and there are no significant consequences. If I make a mistake it doesn't really matter but if I make a good job of it the end result will be there to admire for weeks.'

'I sat on a bench in the garden, in the sun, painting my finger nails in a gloriously decadent shade of red. I know of no more relaxing activity. You have to concentrate totally. It is impossible to think of anything else. Painting your nails requires every ounce of available concentration – particularly when you are using your non dominant hand to paint the nails of your dominant hand. I understand at last why receptionists never even look up when they're painting their nails.'

'Women have the freedom to wear clothes to match their moods. Most of the time men have only the freedom to wear a different coloured tie.'

'I think that transvestites are probably healthier – and may live longer – than non-transvestites. My guess is that transvestites probably suffer far less from stress related diseases than do than do non transvestites.'

'There is a woman in every man. But some men just never let her out. I think they are the unlucky ones.'

'Being a transvestite has caused me a great deal of heartache. But the day I became one was one of the most important days of my life. The day I helped the secret woman in my life to gain her freedom was the day I became a whole man – and the day I found my freedom too.'

'I like the feel of women's underwear. It is softer and more feminine than male underwear and more comfortable.'

'In times of stress and anxiety I need the feel of women's clothing to try and 'escape' from the source of stress. It helps me forget the outside causes of the stress.'

'My cross dressing started when I put on a girlfriend's underwear for fun when we were making love. I liked the feel of it and kept it on afterwards. It made me feel good. My transvestism just progressed from there.'

'I went to an all-boys school and I first dressed as a woman when I was in the school drama society. My voice broke late and I had a rather feminine sort of face so I always got given the female parts. I enjoyed dressing up in silky, feminine things and just carried on. I haven't acted for years but I still wear women's clothes.'

'I put on a girlfriend's teddy when I lost a bet. I had to wear it all day. When I got up the next morning I realised I wanted to wear it again. That was how I got hooked. It was as simple as that.'

'Looking through a clothes catalogue I realised that I was looking at the women's clothes far more than the men's clothes. And it wasn't the models I was looking at – it was the clothes.'

'It is alright for women to dress in men's type of clothing but it is strange that men are considered 'odd' if they like women's style clothing.'

'I have tried to stop wearing 'women's' underwear for various periods of time but have had only limited success. The urge/desire always returns and cannot be controlled. I have explained this to my wife but I do not know if she can understand this.'

'Transvestism is a hobby but it is addictive like drinking, gambling, smoking and the like, but with one major difference – it doesn't kill. But it can hurt, especially if it is your partner or family who finds out.'

'Being a transvestite is the most painful experience of my life. I feel that there is another person inside of me, a female who will not stop at anything to get out. I seem to be more vulnerable when I have had a few drinks. Then she likes to try and take over. I know that it sounds crazy but I honestly feel that this is the case. The agony can drive you mental. The thought of wanting to be a woman, the softness of her clothes, the freedom of her legs; not an hour of the day goes by without this mental anguish. I have tried to suppress my desires but it's almost as if she will claw at my insides to get out.'

'I must say I get a great pleasure and buzz out of dressing up in women's underwear and dresses, getting all made up and putting on my high heels so I can pose in front of my mirrors. I find it so natural to do this and I see nothing wrong in doing so.'

'Why is it that I cannot stop a thing I started sometime in 1976 – the compulsion to wear female clothing and sometimes even make up?'

'I still cannot give it up. I think I'll go on forever like this because I enjoy it so much.'

'I love the feel of silks and satins and wearing silky undies definitely gives me a kick. I am quite able to deal with stress without dressing up and I have no desire whatsoever to be a woman.'

'I know one or two transvestites who blame their parents. They blame their mothers for forcing them to wear girls' clothes and they blame their fathers for not stopping them. I don't see why it's necessary to blame anyone. Transvestism is nothing to worry about and nothing to be ashamed of. It's just something I enjoy. It's great fun. And I love meeting and talking to other transvestites – they are very nice people.'

'The last time I wore any woman's clothing was probably about seven or eight months ago (knickers only). I keep hoping that the feelings will go away and that perhaps the longer I go without women's clothing then perhaps I will be 'cured' of transvestism but this does not seemed to have stopped me looking in the windows of clothes shops and through the women' sections of mail order catalogues and longing to wear the items that I see.'

'I feel the need to wear silky directoire knickers and French knickers. I would also like to wear a silky slip and a dress. Am I cracking up?'

'I suffer very high blood pressure but when I am dressed all the stress and tension goes, and it's a great help to me.'

'I feel as though I am possessed.'

'I used to get sexually aroused, then, not now. Dressing up, for me is as normal as it would be for a woman. I like the touch and feel of clothes – the tight elastic of a girdle, the softness of a pair of tights – there is so much more 'freedom' in a skirt than in trousers or jeans.'

'As I became older and the effects of my war time injuries became much more life threatening the yearning to wear female clothes and indeed to look like and feel like a woman became unbearable. I started wearing female clothes under my male attire and in the evenings would change and put on make-up. This evolved slowly until I had acquired all the skills of make-up and dress sense.'

'There is one great saving grace about transvestism, and that is 'it's the greatest pain killer I know'. Since I have to put up with a great deal of discomfort and pain due to my injuries, I find that I completely and genuinely forget all my pain and troubles when I am 'dressed'.'

'I do it because I enjoy it, feel relaxed and able to calm down, love the feeling of the clothes and give the impression of a woman and sometimes get a sexual kick out of it but not every time.'

'I now find that when I get uptight, just by letting my female persona take over and getting appropriately dressed, the tensions fade.'

'I get enjoyment from wearing feminine clothes. It helps me to relax and allows me to change my character and male image. XX years in the RAF and supposed leader of men – it is great to get away from it, even for an hour or two.'

'I also think it helps me in my work as I have feminine feelings and can talk to all the females working for me and in some way appreciate how hard they have to work to get recognition in a male dominated workforce.'

'I am a happy man. I just like acting the part of a woman. It is relaxing.'

'I always find myself relaxed after dressing up.'

'I enjoy dressing as a woman as it helps to release stress and I like the feelings of dressing and being dressed.'

'I am a serving police officer in the YY Police and after a tour of weekend violence, dressing up helps me to calm down.'

'Instead of reaching for booze or drugs, I reach out for my skirt and blouse and find it far more relaxing.'

'I love women so much that I enjoy dressing like one.'

'I am fascinated by all the paraphernalia of womanhood – garter belts, bras, corsets and so on. I love touching them and wearing them.'

'I don't have to cross-dress. I discovered the art and pleasure of cross-dressing by accident. I do it because it helps me to relax and I enjoy it. What's the big deal? What does it matter to anyone else whether I wear underpants or ladies knickers? It's what inside and what you intend to do with it that counts.'

'Women can have male qualities and still be accepted but men aren't allowed to have female qualities. In my experience men are just as soft as most women – possibly softer. Women think men are hard. But they aren't. Men need sympathy, support, cuddles and reassurance just as much as women.'

'I think of my life in two halves: pre Michelle and post Michelle. (The name I use when I am dressed as a woman). The moment when I first realised I could spend part of my life as a woman was one of the most important in my life.'

'I used to suffer from all sorts of stress symptoms. I had to take tranquillisers and sleeping tablets. Since becoming a transvestite my symptoms have virtually disappeared. I would much rather be a transvestite than a stress sufferer.'

'I used to be a very aggressive workaholic. I was always picking rows with people. Since I became a transvestite I've changed enormously. My wife says I'm more fun and more likeable now. I think I'm an altogether much nicer person.'

3. Survey Results: The incidence of transsexualism among cross-dressers.

Question asked: If you had the opportunity would you have a sex change operation?

23% of respondents answered 'yes'

77% respondents answered 'no'

Commentary

Many lay people who come into contact with transvestites confuse cross dressing with transsexualism. Wives, girlfriends, employers, workmates and friends often suspect that transvestism is merely a stepping stone on a longer journey; a half-way house on the way to transsexualism. This mistaken view is also common among many professionals (doctors, psychologists and social workers) who assume that transvestites and transsexuals are merely variations on the same theme. Some psychiatrists regard cross-dressing as an illness and diagnose transvestites as gender dysphorics but on the evidence obtained by this study I would regard that as nonsense. Some transvestites would like to become transsexuals but most transvestites (over three quarters according to this survey) have no doubts about their gender and are perfectly happy about their cross-dressing. Their problems (if they have any problems) arise almost exclusively from society's reaction to their cross-dressing rather than from their cross-dressing itself. It would be, perhaps, more accurate to describe transvestites as social dysphorics.

'I don't want to be female or have a sex change operation,' wrote one cross-dresser. 'I like dressing up because it brings out the feminine, softer side of my personality and helps me calm down and relax. It helps me to be a more balanced, stable person. Who is nutty? Me? Or the man who smokes too much, drinks too much and takes pills to help him deal with his stress?'

Transvestites and transsexuals themselves often add to the confusion by mixing together and sharing clubs and magazines. They do this because they are brought together by the fact that they are rejected by society. But conflicts often develop. Transsexuals sometimes regard transvestites at 'playing' at being women. Some transvestites, on the other hand, feel uncomfortable with the fact that transsexuals are often sexually attracted to men. To add to the confusion those transvestites who do have homosexual inclinations are frequently attracted to transsexuals.

The fact is, however, that there are differences between the needs and driving forces of many transvestites and the needs and driving forces of transsexuals; a difference made most clear, perhaps, by the fact that transvestism is an exclusively male phenomenon (women do it but since society allows women to dress as men they face no problems or social isolation) whereas transsexualism affects both men and women. Male transsexuals want to be women. Male transvestites want to dress in feminine clothing. There is a huge difference. Many cross-dressers are intrigued and delighted by the paraphernalia of dressing in feminine clothing: stockings, corsets and corselettes, brassieres and so on. Some want to behave like women, look like women and even be treated like women but they do not want to be women. Curiously, when they dress as women, transsexuals often wear jeans or trousers (just as many gender females do) but transvestites nearly always wear frocks or skirts.

Despite the significant differences which do exist between transvestites and transsexuals there is one common area (apart from the important fact that both tend to be attacked, ridiculed, persecuted and subjected to entirely unjustified prejudices): some transvestites (like all transsexuals) admit to a strong desire to have their own breasts. The conflicts here are considerable. Transvestites do not usually want to take hormone therapy (because they know that it will affect their sexual prowess) and they are usually unwilling to consider surgery (because then they would have to share their secret with their family doctor). On top of all this their yearning for breasts is balanced, and to a certain extent overwhelmed, by the fear that breast tissue would almost certainly be impossible to hide from wives, girlfriends, workmates and others. For most transvestites this problem has been solved by the development of new bras which, because they are designed to give an enhanced cleavage to a relatively flat-chested woman, can give a modest cleavage to almost any male. Transvestites who want a bigger bust than can be obtained in this fashion use a variety of techniques ranging from silicone prostheses to heavy duty balloons filled with wallpaper paste. The number of 'she-males' in any community (a she-male' is a transvestite who still has male genitals but who also has breasts – provided by hormones or by surgery or by both) is extremely small. Many young she-males work as prostitutes.

Quotes from cross-dressers

'When I dream of womanhood I see myself as a slender, demure female. I know that even full gender reassignment wouldn't give me this and could possibly lead to an unhappier situation than I'm in now. So for now I'll take my pleasure in stepping into Kate's shoes on a temporary basis.' (Kate is this man's femme name – the name he uses when dressed as a woman. Most transvestites have a femme name.)

'I have no desire to change sex. Escaping from my male body to a female body by having surgery would be a false escape. I would simply take all my old baggage and problems with me. As a transvestite I have the best of both worlds. I can keep all the unpleasant parts of my life in my male world and have the fun as my female self. Being a man isn't about having a penis any more than being a woman is about having a vagina; both are much more than that.'

'I don't want to be a woman but I wish people would understand that some men have many qualities which are generally regarded as being exclusively female. It doesn't seem fair that it is all right for women to have male qualities (ambition, aggression and so on) but it is not acceptable for men to have female qualities. I have a theory that men are just as romantic as women – and probably less inclined to be physical.'

'I love women so much I like to dress like them. That's all.'

'As a transvestite I have had a hard time from straights, gays and transsexuals because I don't fit into any neat category. People get confused. I feel that I am attacked and ridiculed by everyone. I am heterosexual and so gays don't like me. And yet because they think I am gay I'm not accepted by ordinary people.'

'I just love to get dressed as much as I can in women's clothes for I'm a woman in a man's body. I used to have a male boyfriend and he was a smashing and loving fellow and he treated me as woman with love and sex. We were just like husband and wife and were always talking about getting married. But I think we were a bit

23

frightened to go to see anyone about it so in the end he walked out on me.'

'I want to be like a woman but I would not have a sex change operation.'

'Male transsexuals are like golfers: they always lose their balls. Transvestites would run a mile if threatened with the loss of theirs.'

'I would like to be a woman but I don't know if my family would approve.'

'I am living the apparently happy life of a lad who does fancy the girls but would, quite often, rather be one of the girls.'

4. Survey results: extent of cross-dressing

Question asked: Do you dress completely as a woman (e.g. including wig, make-up, etc.)?
76% respondents answered 'yes'
24% respondents answered 'no'

Commentary
Some transvestites wear only female underwear. Some wear only one particular type of female underwear (e.g. panties, slips, stockings and garters). But most go all the way – and dress completely as women.

Most agree that they reached full transvestism slowly and in stages. 'I began by wearing knickers under my trousers. Then I wore a camisole under my shirt as well. After that things just rather snowballed. When I started cross-dressing I never imagined that things would go as far as they have. But I'm very happy.'

Many transvestites, particularly the shorter, smaller ones, buy their clothes direct from women's shops. Some shop themselves while cross-dressed but many shop in their male clothes and explain their purchases by saying that they are buying a present for a woman friend. A few shop in their male clothes and, if questioned, explain to the assistant that they are transvestites. Transvestites often exchange the names and addresses of shops where the assistants are known to be helpful and sympathetic. Some transvestites' wives or girlfriends shop for them. Many transvestites shop in charity shops – partly because prices tend to be lower but mainly because they feel more at ease in shops where male and female clothes are displayed close together.

Those transvestites who do not wish to buy clothing from shops catering to women buy from specialist stores or mail order companies. Many transvestites who buy most of their clothing from the shops women use, also patronise these specialist concerns for the purchase of items such as shoes which may not be available in their size in ordinary stores. (There aren't many high street shoe stores selling high heeled shoes in size 12). The internet has revolutionised shopping for transvestites.

Quotes from cross-dressers
'I do not have the need/urge to dress fully as a woman, it is purely the female underwear which attracts me.'

'I never wear a bra and only put on a girdle or garter belt if I am putting on stockings. I only ever wear blouses, skirts, dresses, knickers and petticoats.'

'I dress as a woman and I do not see why I shouldn't. Lots of women wear male clothing – jeans, trousers, shirts and jumpers. It is sexual discrimination to say that men shouldn't wear feminine clothes.'

'When alone in the house I dress completely as a woman, wearing the nicest lingerie, skirts, blouses, dresses and so on. This makes me feel completely relaxed.'

'I am fascinated by the variety of feminine underwear. Even the words are beautiful. Men wear vests, pants and socks. Women have camisoles, corsets, camiknickers, girdles, garters, knickers, teddies, waspies and a hundred different types of bra: bullet bras, booster bras, balcony bras and so on.'

'Being a transvestite is the ultimate narcissistic experience. I go all the way and make myself look as beautiful as possible!'

'I really do not see what is wrong with a man dressing completely as a woman. In many parts of the Far East transvestites are very highly regarded. In some cultures transvestites were regarded as exceptionally wise and sensitive. The healers and wise men and wise women were often transvestites.'

'I don't believe the differences between the two sexes are anywhere near as profound as some people believe. There is a man in every woman and a woman in every man. Most women have learnt to let their 'male' self out. Transvestites are merely men who are learning to let their 'female' self out.

'I am very particular about how I am dressed when I am en femme. I wear seamed stockings and the seams must be straight.' (En femme is the phrase transvestites often use to describe themselves when cross-dressed).

'Last week I went into a restaurant dressed as a woman. It was my first time. The waiter called me 'madam' throughout my meal and I left him an enormous tip. It was wonderful.'

'I love everything feminine. If I'm feeling down I pop into a store and buy myself some underwear or a pair of earrings. I've got drawers full of stuff but a girl can't have too much underwear or too many earrings, can she?'

'I find that dressing as a woman is a great way to relax. I simply cannot get the same level of relation when dressed in my male clothes. Dressing as a woman provides me with a definitive way of escaping from my male persona – and it brings out the gentle, feminine, non-aggressive side of my personality. When I am fully dressed as a woman I am softer and more easy going. My wife tells me that I am a different person. I find this only works properly when I am fully dressed.'

'It takes me ages to turn into a woman but it is well worthwhile. Shaving is the last male thing I do. I have to shave very carefully to make sure that I don't cut myself. Cuts are very hard to hide and a small nick can ruin a planned evening out.'

'I love dressing up in women's clothes. Male clothes bore me. If you look at paintings of the clothes people used to wear a few hundred years ago you'll find that it was often the men who wore the prettiest clothes. I don't know why things have changed so much. Amongst other animals and birds it is often the male who has the prettiest colours or the most striking plumage. Look at the peacock!'

'I feel that dressing en femme gives me a short cut to another person and another life. I can escape from all the stuff that goes with being a man if I dress completely as a woman. I do the whole thing properly: I shave my chest and paint my toe nails even if I'm wearing a high necked dress and shoes and stockings.'

'Dressing as a woman has given me a real insight into women – and into myself. I discovered that when I am dressed as a man I like to be waited upon because I'm a macho male and when I am dressed as a woman I like to be waited upon because I'm a delicate, very feminine female.'

'I think that the pressure of being a man is much greater than the pressure of being a woman in our society. Dressing as a woman is my way of escaping and so I do it properly.'

'When I dress as a woman I become some quite different. The proof for this claim lies in the fact that when I am a man I never wear anything black. I don't know why but I just don't. I would feel distinctly uncomfortable wearing black. But when I am a woman I often dress in black. I have black dresses and black skirts and I love black underwear.'

'When dressed as a woman I go all the way. I try to feel like a woman as well as look like one. I like to be treated like a woman too. I love being treated gently.'

'I dress completely as a woman and I have learned to be much more sympathetic about the time it takes my girlfriend to get ready when we are going out. I am also more sympathetic about the length of time she spends in the loo! I always use ladies' loos (and sit down to pee partly because it feels right and partly because otherwise it makes a different sound) when I go out dressed and it takes me ages. The first time I went out I put my garter belt straps on over my panties and I was in the loo for ever.'

'Being a transvestite is great fun but you have to be on your toes. I go out dressed quite often and I have to concentrate to remember what sex I'm supposed to be at any one time. I have to remember to remove my nail varnish before people come to dinner, to take my ear rings off when I rush to the door and to put on sensible underpants when I go to the doctor.'

'I sometimes dress completely but I'm sometimes happy to just sit in my frilly underwear watching the television. For me it is the texture which is most important. I've never heard of a transvestite dressing in flannelette, for example. I find frilly, silky things sensual and relaxing.'

'They are only clothes, and you can make yourself as attractive as you like with make-up, and when you feel attractive you feel good. And who doesn't want to feel good in this shitty world.'

'Not all women wear make-up every day – I'll wear it and a wig on average four times a week.'

'Some of the TVs I know like to dress up in wedding dresses etc while I stick to skirts and blouses or a dress.'

'I enjoy wearing a skirt whenever I can but I do not like putting a wig and make up on. I have only put a wig on to go out wearing a skirt because I feel it would be more acceptable to look like a woman when I go out wearing a skirt (or dress). But I have been out for a walk wearing a skirt without a wig on. My wife and I prefer this and if it was more acceptable I would do it more often.'

5. Survey results: The negative social impact of cross-dressing on cross-dressers themselves.

Question asked: Has being a transvestite ever lost you a job or a relationship?

16% respondents answered 'yes'

84% respondents answered 'no'

Commentary

At first sight the low percentage of cross-dressers answering 'yes' to this question seems surprising. It is clear, however, (particularly from the response to Question No 13: Do you live in fear of people finding out that you are a transvestite?) that a very large number of transvestites are extremely secretive about their cross-dressing. These transvestites clearly believe that they would lose jobs or relationships if their secret became common knowledge. Most transvestites would probably prefer to be open about what they do. The secrecy tends to add to the guilt they feel. Many transvestites are also aware that it would be much better to tell their loved ones than to have them find out by accident.

I have no doubt that there is a great deal of prejudice against cross-dressing but the evidence from those transvestites who have been 'open' with those around them suggests that they feel that the fears of what might happen may sometimes be exaggerated.

Transvestites who do decide to 'come out of the closet' face a number of problems. First, they have to decide how to tell those around them about their cross-dressing. Suddenly blurting out the truth ('I like dressing up as a woman') can be shocking and even frightening for the individual who knows little or nothing about transvestism. The wife who is suddenly told that her husband is a transvestite may be frightened that he is also gay or that he plans to have a sex change operation. Her transvestite husband may have had years to come to terms with his cross-dressing. She will need some time too. She will need explanations and reassurance in abundance. She may need to talk to the wives or girlfriends of other transvestites.

Second, transvestites who decide to be open about their cross-dressing have to decide who to tell. Should children be told? Which relatives should be told? Should people at work be told? Should the secret be kept from anyone who might find it difficult to accept? These are personal questions which the transvestite will probably feel that only he can answer.

There is also the problem that it is difficult to know what sort of response to expect. A friend who may seem broadminded may turn out to be heavily prejudiced. A wife who might have been expected to remain loving, loyal and understanding may prove to be so horrified that the relationship never recovers. An admission of cross-dressing may lead to a messy divorce, complicated by the fact that the angry wife and her lawyers may believe that they have a heavy stick with which the transvestite can be beaten into submission.

Some people (including doctors and social workers) who encounter transvestism for the first time assume that a man who dresses in female clothing must be mentally ill.

Here are some comments from transvestites on this subject:

'Psychiatrists talk a lot of rubbish about transvestites. The only transvestites they see are the mentally ill ones. I know scores of transvestites and not one of them has ever seen a psychiatrist. I think we are saner than most other so called 'sane' people.'

'I suspect that most of us would have probably needed psychiatric help if we hadn't discovered cross-dressing.' 'Psychiatrists have no idea why we dress or what we get out of it. The only people they see are the ones who are depressed or anxious for other reasons. There are so many transvestites around that there are bound to be a few who are mentally ill. But well balanced transvestites never see psychiatrists and so for psychiatrists to make judgements about transvestism on the basis of the men they do see is crazy. All the golfers that psychiatrists see are mentally ill but that doesn't mean that all golfers are mentally ill does it?'

Quotes from cross-dressers
'I lost my job when someone told my boss they had seen me in a pub dressed as en femme. I wasn't doing anyone any harm – just having some fun with a couple of other transvestite friends. He called me into his office and said he was letting me go because it had come to his attention that I had been seen dressed as a woman. I asked him whether he was unhappy with my work and he said no but that he couldn't have people like me working for him. If I'd been a train spotter and had spent my weekends standing on draughty platforms collecting numbers he would have thought that quite alright. If I'd been a keen climber and had spent my weekends risking my life by scrambling around on cliffs he would have thought nothing of it. But

because I wear stockings, a bra, a wig and a dress I'm unemployable.'

'It annoys me that my cross-dressing has to be kept secret. I would much rather be open about it. But I dare not risk the consequences. Why people should be so uptight about men wearing frocks I do not know – but they are. What the hell difference does it make what clothes I choose to wear? I realise that society needs some rules. I have to wear a jacket and tie if I want to eat in a smart restaurant, for example. But why should anyone care about what I choose to wear in the privacy of my own home?'

'My fear of the marriage breaking up stopped me telling her earlier in our marriage and my fear of losing her before our marriage stopped me telling her then.'

'Perhaps if I told her earlier, soon after we met, I might have reduced the devastating effect that the revelation of my cross-dressing had on my wife.'

'It must have come as a shock that a person who loves trekking, long distance walking and climbing etc wears 'women's' underwear under 'men's' top clothing.'

'As I'm getting older I'm afraid of getting caught out by my wife and the shame it would bring. I am now feeling full of guilt as though I have betrayed her.'

'It has possibly lost me a job.'

'I've never lost a job because I'm a TV because nobody at work knows.'

'As a serviceman the fear of being found out is very real. They say TVism is common in the service. I have seen many dressed as a woman for fun, but I have yet to meet one as committed as I am.'

6. Survey results: Interpersonal recreational external socialisation in controlled and uncontrolled situations. (Going out and having fun).

Three relevant questions were asked:
i) Do you go out of the house dressed as a woman?
47% respondents answered 'yes'
53% respondents answered 'no'
ii) Do you attend parties or social events with other transvestites?
23% respondents answered 'yes'
77% respondents answered 'no'
iii) Do you ever go shopping dressed as a woman?
21% respondents answered 'yes'
79% respondents answered 'no'

Nearly half of all transvestites venture out of the house in women's clothing. But many – those who are most concerned about being seen – go out at night, after dark and often fairly furtively. They stick to poorly lit streets and avoid crowds. This can clearly be dangerous for it is at night, after dark and in poorly lit streets that muggers and gangs abound. Transvestites who wander around lonely streets are also likely to be arrested for suspected soliciting. Transvestites who venture out at night may be more likely to have their secret exposed – because they end up in hospital or in the local police station.

The number of transvestites who go shopping while cross-dressed is quite high. Obviously, the transvestites who go shopping are usually the ones who are best able to 'pass' as women while en femme. Many shop assistants will readily admit that they regularly serve transvestites and a shop which is known to have sympathetic assistants will often get a growing amount of custom from tall, well-built women with rather large hands and feet.

There is a growing number of clubs of various kinds catering for transvestites – though these are usually situated only in the larger cities or towns but most cross-dressers who wish to socialise do so in pubs and clubs which have a fetish or gay clientele. Although there may be frictions, jealousies and misunderstandings, many transvestites, transsexuals, gays and fetishists get on well together;

all groups being aware that as 'outsiders' they are victims of many unjustified prejudices.

Transvestites who go out in public have to deal with the problem of using ladies' lavatories. It would obviously be impossible for someone wearing a dress, stockings and high heels to go into a gents' lavatory. Most deal with the problem by using ladies' lavatories and being as quick and as discreet as they can be.

Quotes from cross-dressers
'Before I married I used to go to gay pubs and clubs all dressed up because I never used to get any trouble in places like that.'

'I always try to dress as conservatively as possible when I'm going out. I think it is important to dress your age if you want to look convincing. Anyone who goes out looking a drag queen is looking for trouble – and will probably find it.'

'I have not left my house dressed as a woman but have returned to my house when its dark especially after midnight after I have been to Z (a nearby town) for our local TV meetings – having a night out with the rest of us girls and enjoying ourselves very much.'

'I go to TV parties and socials quite a lot. Transvestites are terrific people. We don't have orgies or anything like that. We just dress up, dance a bit, have a drink and sit around and talk.'

'Since going out dressed I have discovered that women get far more smiles than men. It's great fun being a woman. Strange women smile at me when I'm dressed because they do not see me as any threat to them. And men smile at me because they want to get into my knickers.'

'I like mixing with transvestites. They are the nicest people I know. Transvestites are generally compassionate and sensitive people who are slow to judge others. I don't know whether men who become transvestites tend to be more compassionate and sensitive than other men or whether men become compassionate and sensitive because they are transvestites.'

'I go to transvestite parties where I can meet other transvestites because I can really let my hair down. We don't just dress like women – we behave like women too. We giggle and gossip and cuddle each other but there is nothing sexual about it. We're just like a lot of girls on a night out. I have a couple of bitter lemons and I'm as high as a kite. When I get back home I take off my high heels, my knickers, my tights, my bra and my dress, my make-up, my jewellery and my wig and then I start worrying again about the mortgage, the car, the bills and the business. Dressing as a woman is the best way I know of escaping from the pressures of being a man.'

'I have been openly dressing, i.e. actually going out, travelling on public transport, socialising, shopping and many other things that normal women do every day of their lives, for the past two years. Before that I was a closet dresser.'

'I have been more happy and content with life since being able to go out dressed and socialise. The trouble is that society is so narrow-minded.'

'I've been to London to a club there, but travelled from home to the club dressed as a man. When I got to the club I straight away got dressed in women's clothes and had a wonderful evening.'

'I go out dressed – but I only go to a little supermarket at the end of my road as I'm not sure if the man who runs it knows what I am.'

'In the local paper there was a help group for TVs advertised. I rang them up and they told me to come down. I made up a story to my wife that I was going out with my mates. I used to hide my clothes in the wheel well of my car and only bring them into the house when I needed them, so off I went with all my clothes already in my car. When I got there I knocked on a big wooden door, and a rather pretty TV in short black skirt and frilly blouse answered the door in the highest stilettos I'd ever seen. Gorgeous long legs in black stockings the top of which were just showing as he walked up the stairs. He showed me into the changing room where there were men in various stages of undress in various items of women's clothes, some of which you could see were very expensive. I felt a bit shy at first, until one young lad asked if I wanted a hand. I said yes, probably because that was the first word that came out. He was in his early 20s and looked sensational. He started to help me undress with his beautifully manicured red nails. Before long I was completely naked. I was completely seduced and was starting to get aroused when he threw my knickers at me and told me to cover my embarrassment. He then set about transforming me into a stunning female form; wig, make up, bra, knickers, skirt, blouse and high heels. On finishing, he planted a big kiss on my lipsticked lips. It felt greasy but nice. He retouched my lipstick but it was at this point I began to worry whether I was gay, because I had just been kissed by a man in lipstick and thoroughly enjoyed it. He asked me my name. I gave my male name but he said no, your female name. I said I didn't have one, so he called me Angie and introduced me to the group. That was a bit weird as they were all ages and were both strange and wonderful. The young lad tried to put me at ease and constantly passed me comments. He asked me whether I was gay, bi or straight. I don't know why but I said bi. He then made a play, sneaking his hand up my skirt. I then felt I had to get out of that place. I made an excuse and left never to return again. So going to a help group didn't help me.'

'I would love to go shopping but being tall I would be very noticeable and make people look twice.'

7. Survey results: Cross-dressers' realistic, critical self- appraisal of their ability to 'pass' in public. (How convincing are you as a woman?)

Question asked: If you go out cross-dressed, in your opinion, how many of the people who see you are convinced that you are a woman?
a) None
b) A few
c) Most
d) All

30% of respondents reported that no one who saw them would be convinced that they were women
23% of respondents reported that a few of those who saw them would be convinced that they were women
21% respondents reported that most of those who saw them would be convinced that they were women
6% respondents reported that all of those who saw them would be convinced that they were women
(The other 20% reported that they never went out cross-dressed.)

When the results to this question are compared with the results to Question 6 (Do you go out of the house dressed as a woman?) there appears to be some conflict. The apparent conflict is, however, easily explained: many cross-dressers who attend special parties and other social occasions attended only by other cross-dressers do not consider that they go out of their homes cross-dressed because they drive to the party venue in male clothes and change at the venue.

Commentary
Most transvestites are very honest and pragmatic about their attempts to 'pass' as women. Only a small number (6%) believe that they could successfully pass as women in any circumstances. Most accept that they are 'read' by at least some of those with whom they come into contact. (The word 'pass' is commonly used among cross-dressers to define their ability to convince others that they are women rather than men dressed in feminine clothing. The word 'read' is used to define the ability of members of the public to 'see through' the 'disguise'.)

Most transvestites are too tall and too broad shouldered to pass easily as women. Large, and often hairy, hands and large feet don't help. In addition male waists, hips and bottoms are usually the wrong shape (though this problem can, to a certain extent, be resolved by the wearing of suitable corsetry and padding).

In order to 'pass' most transvestites would need to have electrolysis to remove all their facial hair. Most are unwilling to do this because they would then have difficulty in maintaining a presentable male image.

Many transvestites also find it difficult to 'pass' because of their voices, although it is possible to slightly soften the usual, deep male voice by speaking softly and blowing slightly to take the edge of the sounds.

Transvestites also admit that it can take many years to learn the behavioural patterns which make women identifiable. For example, women tend to walk with smaller strides and to sit rather differently to men.

Quotes from cross-dressers
'I would say I'm quite convincing with all my gear on. I'm quite tall at 6 foot and my shoes are size 9 but my corset and false boobs give me an hour glass figure and I'm quite a dab hand with the old make-up which helps a lot.'

'When a transvestite says he can 'pass' I have a suspicion that this means only that the people (s)he meets are nice enough not to say anything and that (s)he has created an image which is, at least, not overtly shocking.'

'People see a woman and assume it is a woman. They don't always check to see whether or not every woman they see is a man dressed as a woman. The person most likely to spot a transvestite is another transvestite. Like most transvestites I'm very good at 'spotting' cross dressers.'

'I try to be as convincing as I can be. I think I am quite good at it. I live alone but my neighbours think I am a couple. They see a man and a woman coming and going into and out of the house and think they are two different people. My next door neighbours invited me round to a meal and told me to bring my lady friend. I had to make an excuse. I feel quite bad about it and I think I will tell them the truth soon.'

'I have no idea whether or not anyone 'reads' me. I simply avoid eye contact with strangers and I never turn round to see if anyone is staring at me. If people want to look – or even laugh – that is up to them.'

'I am 'readable' because I am biggish. But I have seldom had any hassle.'

'The male side of my nature is as far removed from my female side as it would be possible to imagine. Nothing at all, in any way, looks or sounds like the person who sometimes gets herself dressed in the evenings.'

'When made up and out I am not aware of anyone having it worked it out. But when you are in the company of transvestites who are not able to 'pass', you are automatically recognised by the company you are with.'

'I find that if I am dressed smartly and sensibly and am pleasant with people that I am accepted by all sorts.'

8. Survey Results: Bra and panties beneath the suit: the number of cross-dressers who wear women's underwear when dressed in ordinary male clothes.

Question asked: Do you wear women's underwear when you are dressed in ordinary male clothes?
75% respondents answered 'yes'
25% respondents answered 'no'

Commentary
The majority of transvestites regularly wear female underwear underneath their male clothing. Some keep a supply of male underwear for visits to the doctor. A minority of transvestites keep the two parts of their lives quite separate – dressing either entirely as a man or else entirely as a woman.

Quotes from cross-dressers

'I go out of the house with 'women's' underwear under my normal clothes. (This includes tights/stockings, camisole top etc) This is mainly at weekends as I am afraid that if I wore 'women's' underwear to work I would be found out and it would affect my future career and family life.'

'Any man who wears cotton underpants and a string vest when he could be wearing garments made out of lace edged silk or satin (or some cheaper but similarly sensuous material) is denying himself constant tactile delight for the sake of satisfying custom and an anxiety about what people will say if he is knocked down in the street and his secret discovered.'

'I wear lacy underwear and I don't care if anyone knows it. I wear beautiful camisole tops underneath a white shirt for work and I'm sure everyone can see them but I don't care.'

'I go shopping with my wife and family with 'men's clothes on top of 'women's' underwear.'

'I avoid using public conveniences when I am outside as I'm afraid of being found out.'

'I normally wear 'women's underwear 3-5 hours per week day and 12-15 hours on a Saturday and Sunday. If I think I will be caught women's underwear is not worn.'

'I would like to wear 'women's underwear permanently.'

'I find it very strange that most clothing manufacturers do not manufacture soft underwear for men. I normally use women's shops for my clothes.'

'I even take a small set of underwear on holiday but there is always the fear that this will be found.'

'When I've got female underwear on under my outdoor wear I always go and take them off and put my dressing gown on before we go to bed.'

'I often wear undies, bra, garter belt, stockings, panties and waspie, also at times wearing an ankle chain, under my male clothes.'

'It gave me some sort of pleasure walking around at work to think that beneath the male exterior that everyone could see was a pair of turquoise silky knickers.'

'I quite regularly wear knickers and sometimes I'll put on a pair of stockings as well underneath my male clothes.'

'I work in an office. In winter I'll wear tights under my trousers, after all, they are warm, and who likes being cold?'

'I wear female underwear all the time.'

'My wife insists that I wear her underwear all the time.'

'I wear female panties all the time and have worn tights and a bra as well.'

'I never mix man and woman in that way.'

'I wear women's underwear most of the time. I feel good deceiving the general public and some of those I work with, but at the same time I feel guilty at deceiving my friends and family.'

9. Survey results: night-time wear.

Question asked: What do you sleep in?
a) The nude
b) Pyjamas
c) Nightie
37% of respondents said they slept in the nude
18% of respondents said they slept in pyjamas
45% of respondents said they slept in a nightie

Commentary

The low incidence of pyjama wearing among transvestites, and the growing incidence of transvestism suggest that the future for the pyjama industry may be less than rosy. These figures suggest either that many of the transvestites who took part in this survey live alone or that they have understanding partners.

Quotes from cross-dressers
'I sleep in the nude except when I'm working nights. I'll slip on my wife's little black nightie and knickers. I just love the feel of the silk against my skin.'

'The nude; but I have slept in both men's traditional stripy pyjamas and women's satin pyjamas.'

'If I could I would wear women's underwear to sleep in. I only do this if my wife is sleeping in our daughter's room.'

'When she (my wife) goes away I sometimes wear one of her nighties in bed and she knows this.'

'I do have nighties but prefer bra and panties.'

'With two children who stay up late – my main outlet at the moment is wearing a nightie at night spasmodically – usually when I become ratty and moody. If anyone else knew I would be very embarrassed.'

10. Survey results: homosexual experiences among cross-dressers.

Question asked: Have you ever had sex with another man?
20% respondents said 'yes'
80% respondents said 'no'

Commentary
The incidence of any homosexual experience among transvestites (1 in 5) is slightly lower than the incidence of any homosexual experience among non-transvestite heterosexuals (usually regarded as 1 in 3). Most of those transvestites who admitted to having had sex with another man said that their homosexual experiences were

isolated. The incidence of genuine homosexuality and bisexuality among transvestites is considerably less than 1 in 5 and probably close to the normal figure for non-transvestite males of between 5% and 10%.

Most men who cross dress to escape from the stresses in their lives are staunchly heterosexual; some may occasionally fantasise about being picked up and made love to by another man but that is usually simply a part of the pretence of being a woman and not a genuine sexual need or desire.

One side effect of transvestism is that men who are impotent when dressed as men may become potent again when dressed as women – simply because they are more relaxed and more at ease with themselves and the world.

There are a number of significant differences between those transvestites who are homosexual or bisexual and those who are exclusively heterosexual.

Heterosexual transvestites tend to dress to escape from everyday stresses, because they enjoy the feel of women's clothes or, quite simply, because they enjoy looking like women and escaping from their male persona. Many explained that they love women so much that they dress like women as a homage to them. Heterosexual transvestites often tend to disapprove of 'drag queens' and flamboyant, erotically dressed homosexual transvestites who, they feel, tend to make fun of women. Some transvestites get into difficult situations because although they enjoy attracting male attention it is often affection and admiration which they crave – rather than sex. They want to be treated as women emotionally rather than physically.

Homosexual transvestites (who can be subdivided into many subcategories – the most obvious of which are the flamboyant drag queens) frequently admit that they dress for the sexual thrill they get – and to attract male partners. Homosexual transvestites frequently masturbate when they are dressed, often fantasising about a homosexual sexual encounter, and then, overcome by guilt, quickly removing their feminine clothes. In contrast, when heterosexual transvestites indulge in sexual fantasies their fantasies often revolve around real women. (Many heterosexual transvestites have had sexual experiences with female partners while cross dressed. More than half of the transvestites responding to this survey said that they had sex with a woman while cross dressed.)

Quotes from cross-dressers
The survey clearly shows that the majority of transvestites are heterosexual. Most of those respondents who added comments to this part of the survey form made their feelings quite clear:

'I have no desire to sleep with a man. I'm not gay.'

'I know quite a lot of transvestites and none of them are gay. It would be daft for a transvestite to be gay. Gays like men and transvestites like dressing and behaving as women.'

'A friend and I take it in turns to take each other out. He's a transvestite too. One night he will dress and I will take him out. The next time we go out together I'll dress and he will play the part of my male escort. We feel that we are less conspicuous this way. Occasionally we hold hands or put our arms around one another when entering a restaurant or walking along the street but it is only for the sake of appearances and it never goes any further than that.'

'I have to say I am a macho man myself at all other times and cannot abide the thought of sex with another man.'

'Wolf whistles make me feel wonderful. It's nice to know that men fancy me – and that I make a convincing and good looking woman. But that's as far as it goes.'

'I'm not gay – I love women so much I want to dress like them.'

Some respondents did write about homosexual relationships:

'We did enter into a brief sexual relationship, but as I didn't consider myself a homosexual, more part-time heterosexual female, it didn't really work out.'

43

'I once met with another TV and we both dressed up at his house. He masturbated me which at the time I found enjoyable, but it raised questions within myself as to my sexuality. I would not wish to go any further than this and I thought myself to be heterosexual but now I think I may be slightly bisexual. I frequently fantasize about doing it again.'

'I went to a gay club once (while I was dressed). A chap chatted me up. I made excuses after a few drinks that I had to go home. We made a date to see each other. He kissed me goodnight. I never got the nerve to see him again.'

'Whilst cross dressed I have acted out the role of a woman and was attracted to a male. I found I was sexually aroused in a peculiar way, lost my inhibitions, commenced fondling his genitals, progressed to oral and allowed him to finish off by penetrating me. I found performing oral sex quite scintillating.'

11. Survey results: The extent and significance of fear of exposure.

Question asked: Do you live in fear of people finding out that you are a transvestite?
69% of respondents said 'yes'
31% of respondents said 'no'

Commentary
Fear of public exposure is the major anxiety experienced by transvestites. The extent to which transvestites will go to preserve their secret is well illustrated by the fact that one anonymous survey respondent took his completed and untraceable survey form to another town ten miles away before posting it to me. Numerous other transvestites copied out the entire survey form in longhand – and then filled in their answers. They did this, they explained, because they had not dared to cut the survey form out of the newspaper in which it had appeared in case anyone saw what they had done.

The worst problems transvestites face generally involve other men. It is male colleagues and friends who are most likely to respond with horror, abuse or disgust when a man is exposed as a transvestite. It is possibly the same men who object to homosexuality and who, through ignorance assume that a man who is a transvestite must also be a homosexual.

The fear that what they are doing is wrong – and would not be tolerated by those around them – means that many transvestites suffer enormously from guilt. Indeed, the extent of their guilt is so great that in many cases it must very nearly match the stress relief they obtain.

In order to help themselves deal with this guilt it is common for transvestites to fantasise about having been 'forced' to dress in women's clothing. These fantasies can sometimes be extremely complicated and sophisticated but the basic premise is simple enough: the transvestite is kidnapped, captured or taken prisoner by one or more women and then coerced, blackmailed or physically forced into dressing as a woman. The person or persons forcing the transvestite to cross-dress is or are invariably female. While cross-dressed the transvestite may be humiliated and often forced to act as a maidservant. This fantasy is particularly common among transvestites who were dressed as girls by their mothers when they were young boys and later told off by their mother, wife or some other relative for continuing the cross-dressing.

Fantasising about forced cross-dressing also occurs among those transvestites who have an added layer of guilt because while they are dressed they enjoy homosexual fantasies. As I have already shown homosexuality among transvestites is no more common than it is among non-transvestites and this type of fantasy is, therefore, much less common.

There is a final, small, corollary to all this: a few transvestites have expressed the fear that if cross dressing becomes more acceptable, more mainstream, their enjoyment may be diminished. It appears that, for a few transvestites, the fact that what they do is secret and forbidden provides some of the attraction.

Quotes from cross-dressers
'I live in fear of being found out by our daughter, work colleagues and family etc. My parents found out when I was about 15, when they found women's underwear hidden within the bed base. They

said it was not normal and confiscated the clothing. They threatened me with calling in a psychologist and I lived in fear of this.'

'I get annoyed about the way people make judgements about people according to the clothes they wear and their general appearance. Such things are trivial and insignificant. It is the inner person that is important. Identity is not about sex or anything physical but is spiritual.'

'A few years ago I decided I was going to be honest about being a transvestite. I was threatened with blackmail by a former girlfriend and I decided that whatever the cost I was going to come out of the closet. I expected to lose work (I run my own business in a small town) and I thought I might lose some friends but I felt that being honest and open was more important. I also wanted to make it clear to other transvestites that they should not be ashamed of what they do. After all, what the hell does it matter in the general scheme of things? I simply cannot understand why some wives get so uptight when they find out that their husbands like wearing bras and panties. In the end I was very pleasantly surprised: I didn't lose any work and instead of losing friends I gained new friends and, I think, eventually ended up with more respect from the friends I have. Most of the women I know were intensely curious about my transvestism – they wanted to know all the details such as whether or not I shave my legs and chest and what sort of make-up I use to cover up my beard area.'

'I live in fear of my doctor finding out and maybe taking our daughter away from us.'

'My wife discovered my transvestism after X years of marriage. This was the result of my wife opening my briefcase one evening. I immediately got into the car and drove to an isolated location to try and commit suicide by carbon monoxide poisoning.'

'I'm not afraid of being found out. Nearly everyone knows about me.'

'I don't often wear women's underwear when we go out in the car because I'm afraid of an accident and that someone will find out what I'm wearing under my clothes.'

'Thank you for listening to me and I'm sorry about the writing but I'm so nervous. You're the first person I've told about what I like to wear.'

'I have been in a steady relationship with the same girl for 7 years and we have been living together for nearly 4 years. About 18 months ago we had a fairly major bust-up and at the time I became frightened that if she found my secret stash of female clothing the relationship would break up permanently. I instantly threw out most of my clothing (a decision I now regret.)'

'I love cross dressing and feel completely at peace with myself while I'm doing it. I myself feel no guilt and would openly wear women's clothes most of the time if it would not be for the hell most people would put my wife and children through. So I choose to stay 'closeted' because it's easiest.'

'As long as you have a fun adult attitude, and don't dress like a whore in public (when shopping and so on), most of the general public take you as you are or (just think you) slightly barmy.'

'I hate it being in me sometimes, the fear of being found out by friends, family, children; the sheer frustration at not being able to dress up at times when I get the desire. There have been a lot of times when I have just taken to cutting myself on my arm (I have between 50-60 scars) because of the frustration and hate of this problem being in me. I just wish a lot more people could understand this problem (especially my wife) and realise that we are not gay and love the opposite sex as much as anyone else. It's just that we need this release from everyday pressures, and dressing up certainly helps relieve stress.'

'Now and again at the weekends I'll spend all day dressed up. If anyone rings the doorbell, I have to pretend I'm not in – obviously!'

'Keeping it a secret is hard work – it makes it seem as if you're keeping hidden some terrible secret – but that's the way it's got to be.'

'Maybe one day it'll be different – but that's up to the general public.'

'If I hadn't got married and had children I would have committed suicide years ago as in today's society I am termed as a freak.'

'I have a great fear of being 'found out' and would do almost to prevent that happening. My wife (we are great pals) does not like it! She puts up with my habit and will help me if I ask her...though she does not like it and for heaven's sake who could blame her?'

'I don't live in fear of being found out as a transvestite as I feel as soon as everybody knows I will be able to do it openly.'

'This took a couple of days as I posted it away from the place where I work as someone may find out. I am glad you did this survey as I'm glad to tell someone albeit anonymously, about my transvestism.'

'I'm not a bad husband. I don't go out drinking, womanising etc. Dressing up was my only vice.'

'This is the first time I have ever admitted being a TV (albeit anonymously).'

'I am completely open about my transvestism and am accepted by my family and workmates.'

'I would leave this town if I was ever found out about my cross dressing. I was nearly caught once and I'm very careful now not to get found out.'

'I bet there are lots of blokes who have these tendencies but are well in the closet to save embarrassment.'

'I do live in fear of being found out. It is still seen as not acceptable to be a TV and could not face the ridicule and rejection that I'm sure it would bring.'

12. Survey results: cross-dressers' experience of the law.

Question asked: Has cross-dressing ever got you into trouble with the law?
4% of respondents answered 'yes'
96% of respondents answered 'no'

Commentary
Although some transvestites report having been hounded and harassed by the police most transvestites (even those who regularly go out shopping or otherwise mixing in the community) have never had any contact with the police while dressed.

Surprisingly, perhaps, several transvestites who said that they had been stopped by the police (usually while driving) said that one of the policemen who had stopped them had later asked them out. Since most policemen work in pairs this contact had usually occurred the day after. The majority of those who reported being asked out by policemen said that the policeman had asked for their telephone number and had rung the next day to ask for a date. This may be fantasy/wishful thinking but there must be a large number of policemen who are gay but who find it difficult to find partners because of their fear of exposure. Finding a male transvestite, whom they could safely assume would be secretive and discrete, and might often wrongly assume to be homosexual, might be regarded by some police officers as a tremendous opportunity.

Many transvestites claim that their fear of the law (and of having an accident while dressed) means that they drive much more carefully than other men.

'We should get lower motor car insurance than other motorists,' wrote one. 'Because I always wear female underwear I always drive cautiously but when I'm fully dressed en femme I always obey the speed limits and other road traffic laws.'

'Transvestites are the safest drivers in the world,' said another. 'I would much rather travel with another transvestite than with anyone else. They take far fewer risks because they don't want to be arrested or to be found in an accident wearing ladies panties and with their toe nails painted red.'

Quotes from cross-dressers
'I have been stopped for potential (and un-pursued) traffic offenses a couple of times when dressed but have received only courtesy from police to date; I always tell them I am a cross-dresser immediately.'

'We did go out only once last year late at night for a walk – 11.30 dressed up. It was bliss! But we haven't done it since. We are afraid we may meet a neighbour or get stopped by the police!'

'It would be a nightmare to get into trouble with the law with regards to my cross dressing.'

'Once I was stopped in my car dressed up by the police. All my documents were correct. In fact the officer asked me for a date knowing I was a TV.'

'I was stopped by a policeman while I was driving and dressed en femme. I had to tell him my real name (though I'm honest enough with myself to suspect that he had guessed that all was not what it seemed) but when he took down my details he also asked for my telephone number. The next day he rang up and asked me out. I assume he must have been gay. Part of me wanted to say 'yes' but I said 'no'. I've regretted it ever since.'

'I have not yet had trouble with the law because I always go out in the dark and avoid crowded places. If I go out in the daytime I go out in the car. I may try going to a gay club used by TVs.'

13. Survey results: sexual experience of transvestites while cross-dressed.

Question asked: Have you ever had sex with a woman while you've been dressed as a woman?

55% of respondents answered 'yes'
45% of respondents answered 'no'

Commentary
The number of transvestites who have made love to their wives, or girlfriends, while cross-dressed will probably surprise many – particularly those who, quite wrongly, assume that transvestites are gay. The fact that over half of the survey respondents said that they had sex with a woman while 'dressed' also shows that many women do accept transvestism – and enjoy their partner's dressing.

Quotes from cross-dressers
'If you've never been fondled through silk you've never been fondled.'

'My wife makes me dress in a black or red slip, bra, panties and stockings on alternate nights. She loves to fondle me for 30-45 minutes, slipping her hand over the slinky underwear. This gives her an orgasm. Then she sits astride me and quickly has another.'

'There is no doubt that some women are really turned on by making love to transvestites. They call us 'dicks in knickers' or 'cocks in frocks'.'

'I love being caressed through sexy underwear. And my wife loves it too.'

'I would like to, but I doubt if my wife would agree and I accept our unspoken understanding.'

'I would love to wear a pair of silk panties in front of my wife and have her masturbate me but I'm afraid this will never be.'

14. Survey results: Female partners' attitudes towards cross-dressing males.

Three relevant questions were asked:
i) Does your (female) partner know of your transvestism?
74% of respondents answered 'yes'

26% of respondents answered 'no'
ii) Does she approve?
43% of respondents answered 'yes'
57% of respondents answered 'no'
iii) Does your partner help you choose clothes, make up etc?
37% of respondents answered 'yes'
63% of respondents answered 'no'

Commentary

Wives and girlfriends who know that the men in the lives cross-dress respond in many different ways.

At the one extreme are the women who are disgusted by the very idea of a man putting on a woman's clothes. If they tolerate it at all they do so with a bad grace and with very strict rules. Their partners are allowed to dress only at certain times of the week, only in certain rooms and always behind locked doors and with the curtains drawn.

At the other extreme there are the women who enjoy their partners' transvestism, who share their partners' pleasure and who see it as adding to their relationship.

In between there are as many shades of acceptance as there are relationships.

Quotes from cross-dressers

'I worry my wife will find out about my cross dressing because she would divorce me. I wish we could talk about it and be open about it but she just wouldn't understand me.'

'My partner does not have a clue that I'm a transvestite.'

'I started to wear women's clothes when I was about seven years old. Looking back, I think I was always aware of not feeling quite right dressed as a boy. I would dress up in my sister's clothes whenever I had an opportunity, but it would always be my secret. As the years went on I continued to wear women's clothes but always in private, and with a sense of guilt. I got married and my wife and I had three children. I thought that I could get over my cross dressing but it was impossible. So I told my wife all about it. She was very shocked of course, but she is such a wonderful person and tries to help me in all ways.'

'This was a major reason why I did not get married until I was about thirty.'

'All my girlfriends have lot of fun with the TV stuff.'

'She accepted my position of dressing when we were first married (married 23 years) but recently she has changed her position. She still knows I dress up.'

'My wife doesn't approve at all but the transvestite group I'm a member of is run by a woman (we call gender females 'real girls'). I find that this makes me feel more comfortable than if the organisation was run by a man, partly because I am definitely heterosexual and partly because it is comforting to know that not all women reject us as perverts. To know that there is at least one woman who accepts and understands and doesn't judge is very important.'

'My partner knows that I wear this sort of stuff and I've even got some of her cast-offs. She doesn't encourage or discourage me. She just says that I'm not hurting anybody but she doesn't like to see me in them.'

'(My wife was) totally against for our nearly 40 years of marriage until the last 3 months when she started buying me underwear. That's how I know she knew she was going to die and tried to make me happy before she left me.'

'I have tried talking to her about men who wear women's panties to which she said they are queer. I've also dropped hints at Christmas that I would like silk boxer shorts to which she called me a silly old fool.'

'In the main my wife puts up with my transvestism and will accompany me on nights out in the winter while on other instances she will deliberately put obstacles in my way knowing I intend to dress up on that particular day.'

'In my experience it is usually only men who disapprove of transvestism. Women understand that wearing nice clothes does make a difference to the way you feel. I have told dozens of people about my transvestism and the only people who have ever made a big thing about it have been men.'

'My girlfriend was really surprised when I told her. She said afterwards that she had known I wanted to get into her knickers but that she hadn't realised that I wanted to get into her knickers literally – and to keep them on! She thought it was a real laugh and has been great about it.'

'In shops my wife and I compete to find the prettiest bras in our sizes.'

'Although my wife does not approve, she does give me her discarded underwear.'

'We both have found that the first rule of being accepted as we are is to be honest with everyone. That way they have the choice of either walking away or mixing with us socially. Not many walk away. Women do find us fascinating and want to know all about us and although being a transvestite does not lend itself to long-term relationships neither of us is ever short of female company.' (From a letter from two transvestites).

'When I met my present wife B years ago she was happy to go along with dressing me up, saying she regarded it as a game, but after C children and D years of marriage she decided she hated it, saying she thought that I would grow out of it as I got older.'

'I'd like to find a partner who understands and accepts my cross dressing. Transvestites have a tremendous amount of respect for women – after all we dress as them – loyal, caring, loving; it's all there, if a woman wants it.'

'My wife says that what I do cannot be natural since I am so secretive about it. And yet she won't let me tell anyone because she says that I would lose my job and my position in society if it became common knowledge that I am a transvestite.'

'Compliments are like music to the transvestite and she may well seek them just like any woman. My wife is marvellous that way.'

'My wife has helped a little with buying some clothes and selected my female glasses.'

'Quite often dresses and blouses tend to fit us both.'

'One night she was out and her mother had sent down a bag of dresses etc for a jumble sale. As I was fed up I 'borrowed' panties, stockings and girdle from my wife's cupboard and tried on a silky dress which fitted me perfectly. My wife came home early and caught me. From then on, every Saturday night I was her 'maid', washing, ironing etc with full make up. This lasted for about four years and then abruptly stopped.'

'Eventually I set my camera timer up and took a photo of my bottom half in short skirt, stockings and high heels, and I left the photo in the phone book for my wife to find. At first she was convinced it was of another woman, but I told her it was me. She went berserk, she was going to leave, she burnt all her underwear and replaced it all with dull unattractive stuff. She cried for about a month and has totally banned any talk of it in the house. If anything appears on the television or in the papers, she goes into a decline about it.'

'It was my only secret from her and I feel I should have kept it.'

'After telling my wife we went through all the usual nightmares until I was able to convince her that I was not gay etc.'

'I have no partner – but both sisters know and approve.'

'Also any of her friends who stayed here, well if the opportunity arose, I'd be into their kit. I must have tried on the clothes of about 20 or more different women, all without them having a clue.'

'Since my wife found out I cross dressed she has been a tower of strength, advising with my clothes, make up etc. It has brought us closer.'

'The reason for the PO Box is I don't want my wife to find out I am a transvestite. I would like her to know because I would like someone to help me buy clothes, make up etc and help me to dress up properly, but I also wouldn't like my wife to know because I love her and she might not understand me being a transvestite and I don't want to risk my marriage.

'Late wife knew about my desire but could not accept it. Only dressed in secret, subject was never mentioned again between us.'

'My wife likes me dressing. She says I become softer and more feminine when I am changed.'

'My daughter helps me.'

'She does her best and says that it is OK for me to cross dress. Her main concern is that I am not found out.'

'She buys, I try.'

15. Survey results: Hours a week spent cross-dressed: reality and expectation.

Two relevant questions were asked:
i) How many daytime hours a week do you spend dressed as a woman?
The average response was 12 hours (range: 0 hours to 168 hours)
ii) How many daytime hours a week would you like to spend dressed as a woman?
The average response was 70 hours (range: 1 hour to 168 hours)

Commentary

It is here that the difference between transvestites and transsexuals becomes most obvious. Whereas transsexuals say (by definition) that they would like to spend 168 hours a week as a woman the majority of transvestites are keen to retain their mix and match approach to sexuality. Although most transvestites would like to be able to spend more time 'dressed', and the vast majority of those who are still 'in the closet' would like to come out into the open, nearly all of the transvestites who took part in this survey made it quite clear that they did not want to stop dressing as men. For most transvestites cross dressing is a part of being male – not an alternative.

Quotes from cross-dressers
'The skeleton in my closet wears silk panties, ten denier stockings and an itsy bitsy satin bra but that doesn't mean that I don't still enjoy male things. I still watch football and mess with my car like any other man.'

'If it was possible – (I'd cross-dress) most of the time.'

'All the time if I felt in the mood. But I still enjoy my male self.'

'Probably 30-70 hours. But I also have a male existence which I also enjoy at work, in sport and as a TV I can have much of the best of both worlds – male and female. I don't mix the two. I am either one or the other!'

'This is a hard one to answer as I feel if you did it too often, the feelings of enjoyment would be reduced or disappear altogether.'

'I spend most of the weekend dressed, or as much as possible.'

'I would dearly love to enjoy the same freedom as women who wear trousers and jackets without fear of public condemnation or arrest. Probably the only way that this innocent behaviour will ever be tolerated is for it to become fashionable.'

'I would like to wear a skirt or dress most of the time if I could, but I do not like wearing a wig or make up.'

'At present I manage to dress for approximately 10 hours a week but like all TVs I would dress all the time if society would accept it and I wasn't persecuted, made a laughing stock and was accepted for who I am and what I know.'

'(I dress) three hours a night, seven nights a week. We are retired, having sex morning and afternoon. But I've been known to dress up early.'

General conclusion

In recent decades, women have quite reasonably claimed the right to do nearly all the things that men do – and to behave in many traditionally 'male' ways. Women now fight fires, drive lorries, sit in the boss's chair and exhibit emotions which were traditionally regarded as male – and which, in the past, women usually had to suppress. Women can be as tough and as aggressive as men without anyone thinking any the worse of them. And they can wear male clothing without anyone batting an eyelid.

But while women have won the right to exhibit qualities which used to be regarded as 'male', most men still don't feel able to exhibit traditionally female qualities.

Although they now have to cope with a world in which women's rights and expectations have changed, most men still hide their emotions from one another, and from themselves.

At heart most men are just as romantic, compassionate and sensitive as most women. (Indeed, research shows that women tend to be much stronger and more capable of dealing with divorce, unemployment and bereavement than men are.) But those basic feelings are often suppressed.

A surprisingly large number of men dare not admit their femininity to themselves – let alone show it to others. Natural feelings are suppressed and bottled up and, as a direct result, men suffer from high blood pressure, heart disease and immune system disorders.

While women have enlarged their role in society (and have, as a result benefitted in many ways) men have been pushed further and further into their destructive and damaging masculinity.

The old fashioned theory that men are men, that women are women and that, in addition to the obvious physical differences, there are fundamental physiological and psychological differences which mean that men and women see the world through entirely different eyes and must, in consequence, respond entirely differently to identical stimuli, is a nonsense. The theory no longer applies to women but still applies to men.

Society has tried to define males and females in harsh black and white tones whereas in reality the truth is that people exist in a vast variety of shades of grey.

It seems that transvestism provides for many men a healthy release of feelings which would otherwise have remained hidden.

Cross-dressing has been described as a 'symbolic excursion across gender boundaries'. It is probably a healthier and more natural excursion than we realise for it enables a man to show his 'softer side'. And it seems reasonable that men should have the right to express their femininity, in just the same way that women have fought for and won the right to express their masculine qualities.

Men should not be ashamed to show their female qualities; they should not be reluctant to let their emotions show, to ask for help and support, and to combine traditional male toughness with the soft, gentle qualities which are hidden deep inside.

And women should do their best to encourage their men to show their femininity. These days it isn't women who need liberating but men.

There are many practical ways in which men can let their soft, feminine nature surface. They can learn to share their fears and admit to their vulnerability; they can learn to listen to their instincts more often and they can share their feelings with friends.

But it isn't always easy to do these things when you've spent decades doing the opposite.

And so increasing numbers of men are finding that there is a short cut: by dressing in soft, feminine fabrics they can quickly liberate their feminine, gentle side – and (temporarily at least) escape from their aggressive, ambitious, demanding masculine selves.

After all, women often dress as men when taking on male attributes. The woman truck driver may wear jeans and a plaid shirt. Many female executives wear smart suits and carry briefcases. Some women hardly ever wear dresses or feminine clothing at all – claiming that they find trousers more comfortable, more practical and more satisfying from a personal point of view.

(As an aside, it seems rather sad that determined feminists, themselves often full-time cross-dressers, are frequently the most vocal critics of male cross-dressing. It seems curious that women who have fought for, and won, the freedom to live their lives as they wish, and the right to dress however they choose, should feel

60

justified in expending effort condemning men who are trying to obtain the same freedom.)

This survey shows that the benefits of cross dressing are great. So many transvestites get stress relief from their cross-dressing that doctors should consider encouraging some of their harassed male patients to try wearing feminine clothing occasionally. As a doctor, I have no doubt that this would be more useful, and far less damaging, than prescribing another ton or two of anxiolytic and antidepressant drugs.

Many people still regard cross dressing as a joke. It is something that often attracts sneers and giggles. And there is no doubt that a good many people find it unnerving and slightly disturbing. But, from a medical point of view, it seems clear that if there were more transvestites in our society there would probably be fewer men suffering from heart disease, cancer, high blood pressure and ulcers. And that's no laughing matter. (There is real evidence that men who cross-dress are often able to reduce their blood pressure to a point where they no longer need medication.)

Sadly, many of those who have found the courage to escape from the stresses of twentieth century life by putting on panties, bra, stockings and a dress still feel guilty about what they do.

It is time for the sneering to stop and the guilt to be banished. Women fighting for liberation often burnt their bras; men fighting for liberation are now wearing theirs.

I was saddened by many of the letters I received while preparing this report. There is nothing wrong with cross-dressing but there is a great deal wrong with a society which deals so harshly with such a modest behavioural variation from the accepted norm. Prejudice, intolerance and fear breed guilt and shame, which lead directly to anxiety, depression and physical illness. What a pity that is, when there is evidence that men who wear bras, panties and dresses may be protecting themselves from serious health problems.

Our society requires many of us to dress up and wear some sort of uniform. The judge wears a gown and a wig. Soldiers, policemen and people who work in supermarkets wear uniforms. Hotel porters, car park attendants, railway staff, airline cabin crew and nurses all wear uniforms. Doctors wear white coats. Plumbers wear overalls. Bishops wear particularly fine gowns. Bankers wear pinstripe suits.

More than ever before in history we define people by what they wear.

Men who dress in clothing usually regarded as being 'feminine' are throwing a spanner into the works of a finely balanced piece of social machinery. So it is, perhaps, hardly surprising that cross-dressing produces confusion, bewilderment and resentment. Dressing up in feminine clothing is one of the most harmless activities imaginable but it is also one of the most socially misunderstood and challenging.

The most important conclusion from this survey is that men who dress in feminine clothing bring out a normal, healthy part of themselves; they broaden their outlook on life, and they enjoy a temporary respite from the responsibilities, demands and expectations associated with being male.

The cost of cross-dressing is small, the real side effects non-existent and the benefits enormous.

Note:

For a list of books by Vernon Coleman, please visit either www.vernoncoleman.com or Vernon Coleman's page on Amazon Author Central.

www.ingramcontent.com/pod-product-compliance
Lightning Source LLC
Chambersburg PA
CBHW032120280326
41933CB00009B/931